# Sex Body Language

The Comprehensive Guide to Nonverbal Sexual Communication and the Art of Nonverbal Seduction/Cues during Sexual Intercourse

Cheryl Bach

# Sex Body Language

Cheryl Bach

# Table of Contents

# 1

# **Introduction**

Sex is an intimate experience that involves more than just physical touch and verbal communication. It also involves nonverbal cues, or body language, that can reveal our desires, preferences, and emotions during sexual activity. Nonverbal communication can be a powerful tool for understanding and exploring our own sexual desires, as well as our partner's.

Nonverbal communication during sex can include things like eye contact, facial expressions, body orientation, touch, and gesture. These cues can indicate pleasure, discomfort, excitement, or even hesitancy. By learning to interpret and respond to these cues effectively, we can enhance our sexual experiences and create more satisfying and fulfilling sexual relationships.

## Importance of Nonverbal Communication during Sex

The importance of nonverbal communication during sex cannot be overstated. In fact, it is often said that communication is the cornerstone of any healthy relationship, sexual or otherwise. When we are able to understand and respond to our partner's nonverbal cues, we can create a sense of trust, intimacy, and vulnerability that can lead to more satisfying and pleasurable sexual experiences.

Nonverbal communication is an important aspect of human interaction, especially during sexual activities. It can play a crucial role in creating and enhancing the intimacy, pleasure, and satisfaction that we experience during sex. The ability to read and respond properly to nonverbal cues during sex could take your sexual experiences to a new level of enjoyment.

One of the primary benefits of nonverbal communication during sex is its ability to create an increased sense of intimacy between partners. When we use nonverbal cues like eye contact, touch, or gestures during sex, it sends a signal to our partner that we are emotionally invested in the experience. This can help to build trust, deepen the connection and create more pleasurable experiences.

Additionally, nonverbal communication during sex can allow partners to communicate their desires or preferences without having to explicitly verbalize them. Sometimes desire might not come out as words, and nonverbal cues can serve as an effective way to communicate our sexual desires. For example, moans or breathing patterns can indicate pleasure, while changes in body movements can signal discomfort or dissatisfaction.

Another benefit of nonverbal communication during sex is that it can help us to better understand and respond to our partner's wants and needs. By paying attention to our partner's nonverbal cues, we can more easily pick up on the ways in which their preferences and moods are changing throughout sexual activities. This allows us to adapt our approach and better satisfy our partner's desires.

Overall, nonverbal communication plays a significant role in sexuality, and ignoring it could prevent you from achieving more enjoyable, meaningful, and satisfying sexual experiences. By being aware of nonverbal cues during sex, learning how to interpret and respond to them effectively, and communicating our own desires through nonverbal cues, we can deepen our connection with our partner and enhance our sexual satisfaction. Moreover, it helps to create a space for open communication without feeling the pressure to verbalize every desire. It is important to note that the effectiveness of nonverbal communication during sex may require practice and patience. With time, you will begin to feel more comfortable picking up on nonverbal cues and utilizing them in meaningful ways during sexual activities. By understanding and utilizing nonverbal communication during sex, you can connect with your partner on a deeper level and create more pleasurable and fulfilling sexual experiences for everyone involved.

## Overview of the Book

Many people struggle with interpreting or expressing nonverbal cues during sex. This can be due to a variety of factors, including cultural differences, past sexual trauma, or social and emotional barriers. That's where this book comes in.

"Sex Body Language: The Comprehensive Guide to Nonverbal Sexual Communication and the Art of Nonverbal Seduction/Cues during Sexual Intercourse" is designed to provide you with an in-depth understanding of nonverbal communication during sex. It will explore the different types of nonverbal cues that may be present during sexual activity, as well as offer tips on how to interpret and respond to these cues.

This book will also cover ways in which you can use nonverbal communication to enhance their sexual experiences. By learning the art of nonverbal seduction and using nonverbal cues to communicate their desires and preferences, you can create a more satisfying and fulfilling sexual experience for both themselves and their partners.

In addition to exploring the importance of nonverbal communication during sex and how to use it effectively, this book will also cover some common barriers that may prevent people from effectively communicating their desires and preferences nonverbally. These can include issues like anxiety, trauma, or simply a lack of knowledge or skill in nonverbal communication.

Ultimately, the goal of this book is to provide you with a comprehensive guide to nonverbal sexual communication that will help them to better understand and navigate their sexuality. Whether you are someone who is just starting to explore your sexual desires, or you are looking to enhance your current sexual experiences, this book has the potential to help you to deepen your understanding of nonverbal communication and its role in sexuality.

Throughout the book, you will find practical tips for improving your ability to read and interpret nonverbal cues, as well as exercises and activities designed to help you practice your communication skills. You will also find guidance on how to use nonverbal communication to enhance your pleasure and that of your partner's during sexual activity.

Sex Body Language

Overall, this book aims to provide you with the tools and knowledge they need to improve their communication skills during sexual activity. By learning more about nonverbal communication and practicing these skills regularly, you can create more fulfilling and satisfying sexual experiences for themselves and their partners.

# II

# Understanding the Basics of Sexual Body Language

Sexual body language refers to the physical cues and expressions that we use during sexual activities to communicate our thoughts, feelings, and desires. While verbal communication can be important, sexual body language is often more powerful and can provide a deeper level of understanding between partners.

There are many different types of nonverbal communication that can occur during sex, including eye contact, facial expressions, body movements, breathing patterns, moans and vocalizations, and touch. These cues can indicate pleasure, interest, discomfort, or dissatisfaction, amongst other things.

It's important to be aware of these different types of nonverbal communication during sex, as they can help us to better understand and respond to our partner's needs. In the absence of verbal communication or guidance, reading and interpreting sexual body language can make all the difference in our sexual experience.

**Types of Nonverbal Communication during Sex**

**Eye Contact**: Eye contact during sex can convey a lot of intensity, passion, and connection between partners. It can signal a desire for intimacy or indicate that a partner is feeling vulnerable or exposed.

Cheryl Bach

**Facial Expressions**: During sexual activities, our facial expressions can communicate our level of pleasure and satisfaction. Smiling, laughing, and making eye contact might show excitement while frowning or grimacing might signal discomfort or pain.

**Body Movements**: Nonverbal cues like body movements can tell us a lot about what our partner is feeling during sexual activities. For example, arching one's back or tilting their pelvis can indicate pleasure, while tensing up or recoiling from touch could show discomfort or dissatisfaction.

**Breathing Patterns**: Changes in breathing patterns during sexual activities can indicate excitement, and the state of arousal for both of the partners. With each breath partner take, it can signify their level of arousal, need for different stimulation, or satisfaction.

**Moans and Vocalizations**: Moans and vocalizations can provide valuable insights into what our partner is experiencing during sex. Soft, low-pitched moans might indicate pleasure, while high-pitched screams could suggest discomfort or pain.

**Touch**: Nonverbal cues like touch can be used to express a range of emotions during sexual activities. For example, holding hands or caressing hair during sex can show intimacy and affection, while a rough or aggressive touch might indicate a different state of mind.

**Importance of Reading Sexual Body Language**

Reading your partner's nonverbal cues during sex can help you to understand their desires and preferences more fully. By paying attention to their body language, you can adapt your approach and respond more effectively to their needs.

Moreover, nonverbal cues like eye contact, facial expressions, and touch can communicate a level of intimacy and emotional connection that words often cannot express. Learning how to interpret these cues and respond effectively can deepen the connection between partners and lead to more pleasurable and fulfilling sexual experiences.

Furthermore, reading and responding to nonverbal cues during sexual activities can also improve communication between partners in non-sexual contexts. Understanding how your partner communicates during sexual activity can help you to better understand their emotional needs and desires, and this ability to communicate beyond words can enhance your relationship beyond the bedroom.

In conclusion, understanding and mastering the art of sexual body language is an important aspect of successful sexual experiences. By paying attention to nonverbal cues like eye contact, facial expressions, body movements, breathing patterns, moans and vocalizations, and touch, we can gain a deeper understanding of our partner's needs, desires, and preferences. Being able to interpret and respond to these nonverbal cues can significantly enhance the intimacy, pleasure, and emotional connection between partners. So, it's worthwhile for everyone to learn and utilize the basics of sexual body language to improve their sex life and ultimately their overall relationships.

# 111

# **Positive Sexual Body Language Cues**

Nonverbal sexual communication can provide valuable insights into what our partner is thinking and feeling during sexual activities. The ways in which we move our body, express through our facial expressions and voice pitch creates an aura of emotions and messages that can drive our partner towards us or away from us. By reading positive sexual body language cues, you can gain an understanding of what your partner desires, and adapt your approach in response.

Sex Body Language

## Reading Eyes, Lips and Facial Expressions

Our eyes are the windows of our soul, and it's been said that they can also reveal our desires. Eye contact during sex can be very intimate and sexually exciting as it can communicate a lot of passion and connection between partners. If your partner looks deeply into your eyes during sexual intercourse, then he/she is probably feeling very close and connected to you. Dilated pupils and intense gaze may suggest that your partner feels very turned on and excited.

Lip biting is another nonverbal cue that indicates desire. When someone bites their lip during sex, it can mean they are overwhelmed with the pleasure and excitement, or they want to signal their desire and attraction towards their partner.

Facial expressions can reveal a lot about what we're experiencing during sexual activities. Smiling, laughing, or making intimate eye contact can indicate excitement and engagement in the moment. Furrowed eyebrows or tensed facial muscles may suggest discomfort or displeasure.

## Interpretation of Movement

Movements such as hands and fingers moving around the body parts also convey nonverbal cues during sexual intercourse. For instance, if your partner is running their fingers through your hair, it could indicate a deep level of affection and intimacy. Hands running all over the body passionately may suggest how turned on or excited they are, while slow, methodical movements might indicate a desire for a more sensual, slow-paced experience.

## Positive Body Language Signals That Someone is Attracted to You

Positive sexual body language cues indicate that someone is attracted to you and interested in experiencing intimate moments with you. Here are some examples:

**Open body language:** An open body posture can communicate that your partner is receptive towards you and open to physical intimacy. They may lean towards you, relax their shoulders and arms, and uncross their legs.

**Mimicking**: If your partner is mimicking your gestures and movements, it can be interpreted as a sign of attraction and interest. It may indicate they are comfortable and want to get closer to you.

**Smiling**: A bright and genuine smile is hard to fake, so if your partner is smiling at you, it's a good sign that they are happy and enjoying their time with you.

**Physical touch and proximity**: If your partner is initiating physical contact, such as brushing against you or touching your arm, it can suggest that they want to be closer to you. The physical touch will create an emotional connection and deepen intimacy.

**Vocalizing pleasure**: Positive audible cues like moaning, sighing, and deep breathing are strong indicators of sexual pleasure. Such signals reinforce the sexual chemistry between couples, elevate the mood and invite for more sexual experimentation.

In conclusion, reading positive sexual body language cues during intimate moments enhances sexual communication, intensifies passion and builds intimacy. Paying attention to these cues can help you know what your partner likes, what their desires and preferences are, and how to make things more pleasurable for them. Positive sexual body language cues include open body language, mimicking, smiling, physical touch and proximity, and vocalizing pleasure. Understanding and interpreting these nonverbal cues can lead to better communication, more satisfying sexual experiences, and may also help to foster a deeper intimate connection with your partner.

# IV

# Negative Sexual Body Language Cues

As important as recognizing positive sexual body language cues is understanding negative nonverbal signals. Many people can be uncomfortable in intimate situations, which could lead to unintended miscommunications. Being able to read your partner's negative sexual body language cues can avoid potential misunderstandings and help make sex a more satisfying experience.

**Techniques for Identifying Negative Body Language and Interpreting Them**

Reading your partner's body language accurately requires you to pay attention to subtle shifts and changes in their physical cues. Here are some ways in which you can identify and interpret negative sexual body language:

**Lack of eye contact:** Avoidance of eye contact might indicate a lack of engagement or shyness, which could be a sign that your partner is feeling uncomfortable with the level of intimacy.

**Tensing up:** When someone tenses up during sex, it might indicate that they are mentally or emotionally withdrawing from the encounter. It can also suggest discomfort or pain.

**Crossing arms or legs**: Crossing arms and legs often signals defensiveness and discomfort, which could indicate that your partner is not comfortable with something that's happening or would like things to slow down.

## Common Negative Body Language Cues and What They Mean

**Looking away**: If your partner avoids eye contact and looks away during intimate moments, it could suggest that they're feeling uneasy or embarrassed.

**Rigidity**: Stiffness or tensing in your partner's body during sex could indicate discomfort, stress, or even physical pain.

**Frowning or grimacing**: Frowning, grimacing, or other facial expressions of discomfort during sexual activity may signal pain, discomfort, or a lack of enjoyment.

**Pushing away or avoiding touch**: If your partner is resisting your touch or trying to physically move away from you, it may indicate that they're experiencing discomfort or feeling overwhelmed. It's important to respect your partner's boundaries and take things slow if they appear hesitant or uncomfortable.

**Lack of responsiveness**: If your partner isn't responding to your advances or seems disengaged during intimacy, it could be a sign that they're feeling disconnected or not interested.

**Closed body language**: Crossed arms, clenched fists, or other signs of closed-off body language can suggest that your partner is feeling guarded, uncomfortable, or defensive.

In conclusion, identifying negative sexual body language cues can be challenging, but it's essential for building trust and intimacy with your partner. Paying attention to subtle shifts in your partner's body language during intimate moments can help you understand their needs, desires, and boundaries and ensure that you are both having a mutually satisfying experience. Remember to respect your partner's body language and communicate openly about any concerns or discomfort you may be feeling in order to establish a safe and pleasurable environment for both of you.

# Sex Body Language

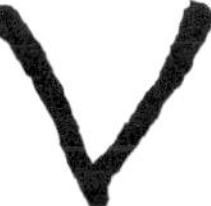

# Conclusion

Sexual intimacy is an essential part of human relationships. It is a physical expression of our deepest desires, emotions and needs, bringing us closer to our partners both physically and emotionally. That being said, communicating these desires, needs, and emotions verbally isn't always feasible, which is where nonverbal sexual communication becomes particularly important.

This book provided comprehensive information on nonverbal sexual communication, including the art of nonverbal seduction and other nonverbal cues during sexual intercourse. We explored the various ways in which people unconsciously use their bodies to express powerful messages during sexual encounters and how to use this knowledge to enhance sexual experiences. The book emphasized that nonverbal communication plays a significant role in sexual intimacy and how paying attention to these cues can significantly improve sexual encounters.

Some of the key insights discussed throughout the book include the importance of reading sexual body language, understanding sexual attraction and desire, increasing intimacy, setting boundaries, and enhancing pleasure during sex. We also explored how cultural contexts can shape the interpretation of nonverbal cues in sexual interactions and the potential impact of power dynamics on nonverbal communication.

Ultimately, this guide provides a comprehensive framework for understanding the complexities of nonverbal sexual communication, which can help individuals foster deeper connections with partners and improve their sexual experiences. By becoming more attuned to nonverbal sexual cues, individuals can communicate their desires, needs, and emotions without relying solely on verbal communication, resulting in more intimate and fulfilling sexual experiences.

Overall, this book highlights how nonverbal communication plays a critical role in sexual encounters and how individuals can use this knowledge to enhance their sexual experiences. It provides practical tips for recognizing, interpreting, and responding to nonverbal cues during intimacy, encouraging readers to enhance their communication skills, build trust, and develop rewarding relationships.

In conclusion, "Sex Body Language: The Comprehensive Guide to Nonverbal Sexual Communication and the Art of Nonverbal Seduction/Cues during Sexual Intercourse" is an excellent resource for anyone interested in improving their understanding of nonverbal communication and enhancing their sexual experiences. Whether you're single or in a relationship, this book offers valuable insights into the art of nonverbal seduction, guiding you to become more skilled in reading and communicating smooth and seamless nonverbal cues that can take your sexual encounters to a whole new level.

9 798321 627358